GET BACK into WHACK

Includes 30-Day Quick-Start Guide and Beyond!

How to Easily **REWIRE YOUR BRAIN** to
Outsmart Stress, Overcome Self-Sabotage,
and *Optimize Healing* from
Fibromyalgia and Chronic Illness

Susan E. Ingebretson

ISBN: 978-0-9843118-6-6

Library of Congress Control Number: 2019914876

Printed in the United States of America
Ordering information https://www.RebuildingWellness.com

Cover Design by 100Covers.com
Interior Design by FormattedBooks.com

NORSEHORSE
PRESS

NorseHorse Press
PO Box 6722
Orange, CA 92863-6722

How healthy is your brain?

Do you wonder if you have an *Out of Whack* brain challenge?

Find out right away.

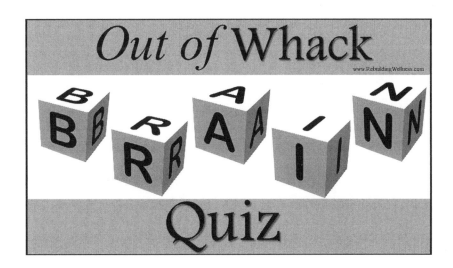

Download your **Brain Quiz & Mini Workbook** now by visiting:

https://rebuildingwellness.com/brain-quiz

PREFACE

....

When I wrote my first non-fiction book, *FibroWHYalgia*, I was quite enamored with the concept that knowledge is power. I learned so much on my healing journey. I discovered the power of nutrition, detoxification, and emotional wellness. I read everything I could find and listened to lectures, watched documentaries, and asked questions of those who knew so much more.

I'm an information sponge.

But that's just me. I love data, and 20 years ago, it was hard to come by. In today's world, we're flooded with it. Over time, I've gathered, gleaned, filtered, and synthesized what I've learned so I can share it. That's my passion.

The great news is that even though I'm thirsty for research, no one expects you to be parched too. In this guide, I've soaked up the statistics on *how* to *Get Back into Whack*, and I've summarized all the critical parts for you.

Things have changed a lot in the past two decades. "Knowledge is power" is still a critical belief — yet it's incomplete. Without application, information alone creates little gain.

> ### *Real traction comes from applying what you learn.*

That's the intention of this workbook. Like a roadmap, follow the themes outlined in the following pages, and you'll arrive at your self-guided destination. You'll reach an objective that's not only different from today but one that's beyond your dreams for tomorrow.

The steps are simple: Grab a pen or pencil, and answer the discovery questions in Section 1 with honesty and curiosity. Then jump into Section 2, and build your plan. By the end of this workbook, you'll have created your life by your own design.

TABLE OF CONTENTS

INTRODUCTION

This workbook has two sections.

The first section features the Head Work questions from chapters 1-18 of my book, *Get Back into Whack*. For ease and simplicity, they're reprinted here with plenty of space to write your views and reflections.

These thought-provoking questions broaden your comprehension of the main principles offered in each chapter. They also allow you the headspace to explore new options and use your sense of imagination and creativity as it applies to problem-solving.

The second section of this workbook features a 30-Day Quick-Start plan to launch your healing journey. Work through the first section of this workbook before jumping into the second. Doing so creates a comprehensive pool of resources to use and apply to your quick-start steps.

This workbook is intentionally kept short and to the point. More information does not always bring more clarity. Yes, *information anxiety,*[1] aka *information overload*[2] is a real thing! Here's a favorite quote on the subject—

---

1   https://www.igi-global.com/dictionary/information-anxiety/38651
2   https://psychcentral.com/blog/overcoming-information-overload/

> ***"We're drowning in information***
> ***while starving for wisdom."***
> — E.O Wilson

Clarity fosters wisdom. Here are a few tips:

- WISDOM comes from applying the information *you* decide is essential.
- WISDOM comes from experience and discernment as you follow your own transformational journey.
- WISDOM comes from knowing yourself so well that you intuitively and innately feel guided in your plan. You confidently follow your "next step" journey most of the time and apply self-compassion and graceful flexibility when you don't.

You'll find it easier to embrace your own 30 days of "next steps" after completing the following Head Work questions.

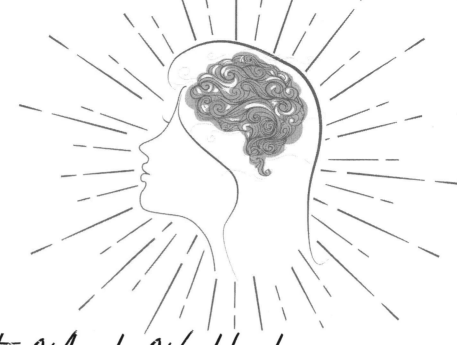

Get Back into Whack Workbook: Chapter Head Work

Chapter 1 – Head Work

1. Review how the limbic system of the brain differs from the cerebral cortex. How does this apply to you and your goals?

Limbic = Emotion   Cerebral = critical thinking.
non-conscious   Conscious – analytical – new data
I naturally observe everything/sense everything especially in places
analyse/judge patterns/cerebral or conscious = limbic so
overwhelmed in place up particular

2. How does your MAPP make things easier for you day-to-day? How might it create limits that aren't so helpful?

My brain is analytical. My outlook is +ve and
compassionate. I am empathic. Think Miss Marple
So aware of others but not self aware.

3. Why is neuroplasticity remarkable when it comes to adopting new habits? For example, if someone considers themselves to be a negative thinker and says, "that's just who I am," does the neuroplasticity principle prove this belief true or false?

Neuroplasticity means you can change your
way of thinking. Nothing is hard wired.

Chapter 2 – Head Work

1. List at least three different circumstances where you've experienced natural brainwave states similar to the state of hypnosis.

    _____

    _____

    _____

    _____

2. What moments allow you to zone out—even if it's just for a bit? Try them out and make them more effective by creating positive intentions while in these states. For example, the last thing before you fall asleep, and the first thing when you wake is a perfect time to implement gratitude and appreciation practices. It's also a great time to set intentions and plans for the success of your day.

    _____

    _____

    _____

    _____

3. Practice paying attention to when and how closed-door thoughts pop into your mind. When this happens, follow up the thought with the three-word phrase shared in this chapter (up until now). See how it shifts your sense of potential.

    _____

    _____

    _____

    _____

Chapter 3 – Head Work

....

1.   Increase your awareness of internal conflicts. What makes you think, "on the one hand…," or "part of me feels…." Notice these conflicts and consider any potential misalignments.

_____

_____

_____

_____

2.   Increase your awareness of behaviors that do not match your plans. Are they sabotaging behaviors? What would you have to believe as true in order for you to stop the sabotage?

_____

_____

_____

_____

3.   Jot down a list of "facts" you believe about your health and your ability to heal. Look for clues that indicate where they may limit you. Can you shift your understanding of these "facts" and instead see them as beliefs?

_____

_____

_____

_____

Chapter 4 – Head Work

1. Have you ever considered the connection between negative thoughts and chronic pain? Explore and list three examples of how your thoughts may transfer to physical consequences.

    _____

    _____

    _____

    _____

2. Awareness begins by paying attention to it. Simply notice your thoughts. (If you feel you don't have self-talk, notice your results. Are they what you want? Pay attention to your patterns of behavior, and you'll soon recognize the thoughts that drive them.) *Notice without judgment.* Make a mental note of your thoughts, feelings, patterns, and reactions to your surroundings. Do you often have knee-jerk reactions? Do you simmer? Do you ignore? Begin to notice and monitor them. Let this awareness percolate a few days and then jot down your discoveries into a journal, notebook, or this workbook.

    _____

    _____

    _____

    _____

3. Do you use self-deprecating humor? Do you deflect comments that make you feel uncomfortable with snarky remarks or put-downs at your own expense? Consider how your reactions are either supportive of your overall goals or how they have the potential to keep you stuck. Brainstorm at least three ways to shift this behavior. Create a personal script for how you'd rather react or respond.

    _____

    _____

    _____

    _____

Chapter 5 – Head Work

....

1. Review your Head Work from Chapter 4. What type of self-talk did you notice when you first became aware?

    _____

    _____

    _____

    _____

2. Write down the basic steps from the Strategies for Dealing with Negative Self-talk found in this chapter. Put them on an index card, notecard, or sticky note. Carry them with you to review often. Which steps come easily, and which are you likely to skip or forget? Practice these steps to make them a smooth and consistent response to negative thoughts. Have you committed to making this change? **Decide** right now to change your response to negative thoughts.

    _____

    _____

    _____

    _____

3. Write down the steps for the FIVE 180 Reset. What happened the first time you tried it? Did you feel a sense of calm right away, or did you have to practice a few times? Keep your written reminder handy so that you follow all five steps. Strategize now for how you'll remember to use this method when stressed. Decide what will make you think of it. (Suggestions: At the first sign of stress in the body—tightened shoulders, stomach in a knot, etc.—practice thinking of a stop sign or a pause button. This initial visual cue can help you to remember this powerful tool. You may even wish to draw or print out photos of stop signs or pause buttons to post as reminders.)

    _____

    _____

    _____

    _____

30-Day Goals Worksheet

(As noted in Chapter 6 of *Get Back into Whack*)

What would you like to achieve in the next 30 days? (Note what you *do* want rather than what you *don't* want). Write down one goal for each of these three categories.

Note this important fact: you're going to create results anyway. You'll either create more of the same results you've already had by doing the same things you've already done. Or you'll set new intentions and make changes in how you think. From there, the actions come as a by-product.

Use a pencil. We'll refine as we go. Or use ink with no worries of scribbles or cross-outs. This is not about perfection. It's also not about creating a finite plan. **Goals are a work in progress**. Life is a work-in-progress.

*TIP: As you work on this list, keep the ADAPT and GROW technique from Chapter 10 in mind. Remember to ask yourself, "Do I want to dabble with my future or commit to doing something about it?" Make that commitment now. List your goals/desires first, and then review the steps in this technique. Look for details that may need assistance or tweaking. Specifically, note areas where you'll need help in defining the amazing **benefits** you'll receive from achieving these goals, the **obstacles** that may seem to be in your way, the **resources** you may need to acquire, and the **support** system you need to enlist.*

Health/Nutrition: _____

_____

_____

_____

_____

_____

On a scale of 1-10 (1 being not at all)—

How strongly do I want to achieve this goal?

1	2	3	4	5	6	7	8	9	10

How much do I believe I have the resources to achieve this goal?

1	2	3	4	5	6	7	8	9	10

How committed am I to this goal? (Notice how commitment is different from wanting.)

1	2	3	4	5	6	7	8	9	10

Self-Growth/Spirituality/Connections: _____

_____

_____

_____

_____

On a scale of 1-10 (1 being not at all)—

How strongly do I want to achieve this goal?

1	2	3	4	5	6	7	8	9	10

How much do I believe I have the resources to achieve this goal?

1	2	3	4	5	6	7	8	9	10

How committed am I to this goal? (Notice how commitment is different from wanting.)

1	2	3	4	5	6	7	8	9	10

Fitness/Body Movement/Activity: _____

_____

_____

_____

_____

_____

On a scale of 1-10 (1 being not at all)—

How strongly do I want to achieve this goal?

1	2	3	4	5	6	7	8	9	10

How much do I believe I have the resources to achieve this goal?

1	2	3	4	5	6	7	8	9	10

How committed am I to this goal? (Notice how commitment is different from wanting.)

1	2	3	4	5	6	7	8	9	10

Chapter 6 – Head Work

1. If you haven't already, go back and write down your goals. Do it now. Fewer than 3% of Americans have written goals.[3] So, beat the odds to proven success and get ahead of the curve. The exact steps to reach your goals will change. They're flexible and fluid, but the intent of the goals themselves stays firm. Outline them here or flip back a page and write/revise.

_____

_____

_____

_____

2. What about the Words to Stumble By mentioned in this chapter? Are you surprised at how often you use them? What about how you use them? Notice how routine (and perhaps habitual) it is to use negative words in relation to your health. Here's an exaggerated example. "I try to get better, but nothing works. I shouldn't eat junk food, but my bad knees hurt no matter what I eat." Notice how many negative references this illustrates? From it, you can hear the sense of helplessness and hopelessness this person feels. From this defeated state, she or he would be unlikely to come up with positive solutions or motivation to change. Our thoughts create the state we live in. How will you choose to create a different state for yourself? How will you *choose* to create an environment that allows more happiness?

_____

_____

_____

_____

---

3   https://www.briantracy.com/blog/personal-success/success-through-goal-setting-part-1-of-3/

3. When it comes to brainwave states, can you think of activities or behaviors that help you get into the Alpha state? What about the Theta state? Brainstorm a few ways to reach these ideal states of relaxation.

_____

_____

_____

_____

Chapter 7 – Head Work

1. What self-sabotaging behaviors came to mind when you read the Spotlight of the Mind Illustration? Did you recognize the gap between something you planned to do and what actually happened? Use this evidence for your benefit. Go back and review your goals listed in Chapter 6. View them from your new understanding of how self-sabotage ensues. Brainstorm ways to overcome or avoid this limiting pattern.

_____

_____

_____

_____

2. Where will you apply SET Switch Motivation first? Write out the steps and review them as you make this method a daily practice.

_____

_____

_____

_____

3. What gateway activities appeal to you most? Consider adding a few to your relaxation practices and experiment. Discover which ones are most effective for you. Of course, feel free to add your own. You're the best judge of what relaxes, soothes, inspires, and invigorates your soul.

_____

_____

_____

_____

Chapter 8 – Head Work

1. Do you relate to my healing story? To what parts? Have you partially recovered from some of your symptoms or eliminated some? Finding the sweet spot of the Restoration Trio can help. What parts of the trio are lacking in your recovery plan? Jot down your discoveries and make changes, if necessary, to your goals listed in this workbook.

_____

_____

_____

_____

2. In what ways does stress add to your pain levels? Does it add to other symptoms too? Be specific as you consider this topic. The effects of stress can be both obvious and disguised. In which of the following areas do you experience the most stress: health, finances, relationships, career, education, personal development, spiritual development, social life?

_____

_____

_____

_____

3. In what ways do you believe your body is inflamed? Read my article, Symptoms of Systemic Dysfunction,[4] and review the signs of inflammation. (You'll find this list as an excerpt in the Appendix of *Get Back into Whack* or read the article from the citation below.) Which ones relate to you? Investigate a few ideas on what areas of your life need focus as it relates to this problem.

_____

_____

_____

_____

---

4   https://www.prohealth.com/library/do-you-have-these-fibromyalgia-symptoms-of-systemic-dysfunction-37277

Chapter 9 – Head Work

1. Review the ways that stress impacts the body. With the polar opposite effect in mind, how do you view your body's reactions? In the past, when you felt stress, what was your go-to behavior? Decide from now on, what your response will be instead.

    _____

    _____

    _____

    _____

2. List three practices you can implement to manage your stress levels.

    _____

    _____

    _____

    _____

3. Plan to implement a deep breathing strategy into your daily life today. Create a micro habit[5] by linking your new deep breathing practice to something you already do daily, such as getting dressed, brushing your teeth, or fastening the seatbelt of your car.

    _____

    _____

    _____

    _____

---

5   https://qz.com/877795/how-to-create-new-good-habits-according-to-stanford-psychologist-b-j-fogg/

Chapter 10 – Head Work

1. What life changes in the past threw you a curveball? Which ones were the most frightening or felt the most threatening? Ponder how you felt when the change initially occurred. Notice, in particular, how you probably could not see the possibilities for benefits from the change. Think about how your thought patterns kept you stuck in the midst of that change. Notice if those thought patterns repeat at other times, even when the change isn't as drastic.

    _____

    _____

    _____

    _____

2. Write down at least three ways that unexpected change has brought you positive results. Consider changes in all areas of life.

    _____

    _____

    _____

    _____

3. Write down the steps of the ADAPT and GROW technique. Brainstorm goals or plans that you'd like to implement using this specific plan. (Review your goals outlined previously in this workbook.) From this list, choose one to implement first.

    _____

    _____

    _____

    _____

Chapter 11 – Head Work

1. After reading this case study, were any of her results unexpected? Did Callie have discoveries or epiphanies that surprised you? Consider that as you implement change, you're often able to see things from a different angle than before you began. What problems would you like to be able to view from a different angle?

    _____

    _____

    _____

    _____

2. Review the problems list you made from the previous question. Write down the steps for the ADAPT and GROW technique. Then consider those steps as they'd apply to the problems you'd like to solve and the goals you'd like to achieve. Choose one and move on to the next question in this chapter's Head Work.

    _____

    _____

    _____

    _____

3. Complete the first two steps of the ADAPT technique in detail. Don't skimp on the time or thought put into this part of the plan. After these steps have been fleshed out, take a moment to consider what comes next. What action steps come to mind first? Don't complicate things by analyzing what's "right" or wondering what may happen down the road. Simply jot down your thoughts and take the next obvious step.

    _____

    _____

    _____

    _____

Chapter 12 – Head Work

1. What phase of the Four Phases of Growth do you find yourself getting stuck in the most? Decide to beat inertia! Implement the Head Work following each chapter and notice how taking action helps to rockyour way out of "stuckness."

_____

_____

_____

_____

2. After reading the Smooth Sailing analogy, what do you think about your "sails?" What choices can you make to harness this part of your health journey? Write down at least three ways you can support your plans through changes in how you think and by shifting to a positive focus.

_____

_____

_____

_____

3. Brainstorm and jot down at least five decisions you can make in advance to reduce decision fatigue. Don't overthink this—keep 'em simple.

_____

_____

_____

_____

Chapter 13 – Head Work

1. Do you tend to have a Negative Nancy in your head? Does that voice shift your focus to the potential for failure? Does it distract you from considering opportunities for success? If your Negative Nancy has anything to say about the potential outcomes of this book so far, jot them down now. Hold off on reviewing this list until after you've read Chapters 14 and 15. For now, just write down your negative thoughts. They need to be heard.

    _____

    _____

    _____

    _____

2. Review the steps provided in the Advanced Strategies and Thought Pattern Review section. All of these steps should be familiar at this point. Identify what step may challenge you the most. Is it noticing your inner self-talk in the first place? Or perhaps it's deciding what you'd rather think instead. Whatever it is, focus on that step in particular and decide to make the solution for it into a habit.

    _____

    _____

    _____

    _____

3. The Change or Chains process is deceptively simple. It doesn't take long to do and putting it into practice can be quite an eye-opener. Each time you find yourself feeling tense, stressed, nervous, or knots in your stomach, reflect on the triggering thoughts. Notice if there's a pattern. Do you often have thoughts that make you feel isolated or alone? What about feeling broken or that you somehow don't measure up? Notice these patterns and choose statements that lead you toward a *changed* future rather than a chained past.

    _____

    _____

    _____

    _____

Chapter 14 – Head Work

1. Review the superpower traits and place an X by the ones you relate to most and believe you already possess (to any degree). Re-read these entries and focus on how they make you feel at a physical level. Engage deeply in the emotions, ideas, and thoughts these traits bring to mind. Notice a deep sense of gratitude as you identify with these traits. Jot down your discoveries.

    _____

    _____

    _____

    _____

2. Review the superpower traits and circle the ones you'd like to develop. Who do they remind you of? What person (known personally to you or publicly known) exemplifies these traits? Write down the characteristics of the person(s) you'd like to emulate. Make a list of the superpower traits you'd like to adopt and review them daily.

    _____

    _____

    _____

    _____

3. Create a visualization practice incorporating your superpower traits. Imagine yourself (employing all senses—sight, sound, touch, smell, taste, AND emotion) deepening your experience with the traits that are familiar to you. View yourself adopting the traits you admire in others and see yourself shifting to think, feel, and act as they do.

    _____

    _____

    _____

    _____

Chapter 15 – Head Work

1. List at least three benefits of implementing a gratitude/appreciation practice. Decide and jot down how you will implement this practice right away.

    _____

    _____

    _____

    _____

2. Which of the three missing traits (happiness, motivation, or willpower) eludes you the most? Using the tips and strategies provided, create a game plan for developing these much-needed emotions and add it to your calendar.

    _____

    _____

    _____

    _____

3. How will you deliberately decide to use your nonconscious mind as an autopilot feature? Success math shows that you'll achieve far more with your internal mental reprogramming than with any other external effort. Which methods appeal to you the most?

    _____

    _____

    _____

    _____

Chapter 16 – Head Work

1. When you think back to your past struggles (whether to heal, change a behavior, or develop new habits), what can you now identify as your biggest hurdle? Was it negative self-talk? Self-sabotage? Limiting beliefs? Identify your common health hurdles and decide on a different path.

    _____

    _____

    _____

    _____

2. Which of the Build-a-Better-Brain practices do you already do? Which ones were completely new to you? Which ones have you decided to implement? Go back and highlight those of interest. Create an outline of your plan here.

    _____

    _____

    _____

    _____

3. Do you have an idea of what tracking method you'd like to put into place? Whether it's plain, fun, colorful, or whimsical, make sure it's simple to do and visually available every day.

    _____

    _____

    _____

    _____

Chapter 17 – Head Work

1. Review the Benefits of the Build-a-Better-Brain list. Highlight those you'd like to achieve most and re-write them here. Notice how the practices you've chosen in Chapter 16 align with these highlighted benefits. Create or revisit your Build-a-Better-Brain practice plan and keep these new benefits in mind.

_____

_____

_____

_____

2. After reviewing the four steps I was willing to take to recover from fibromyalgia, do you notice any that relate to you? Do any of the steps create feelings of resistance? Zero in on any that may pose more of a challenge (possibly steps two and/or three). What actions will you take to overcome or work through these challenges?

_____

_____

_____

_____

3. Review the Daily Healing Recipe offered in this chapter. Write down the key ingredients here and on an index card or sticky note and place it where you'll see it daily. Apply these "ingredients" liberally to your overall health plan.

_____

_____

_____

_____

Chapter 18 – Head Work

1. Which objections or obstacles listed in this chapter resonate with or surprise you the most? Did you feel ownership of it right off the bat, or did you have to sit with it a while? Sometimes objections are clouded by other beliefs, and they may feel only partially true. Sometimes obstacles feel insurmountable. Do a quick internal survey. Notice and acknowledge their presence. Tell yourself you'll address them later if needed. For now, suspend objections that thwart your forward progress and address the obstacles accordingly.

   _____

   _____

   _____

   _____

2. Write down "I don't…" on a sticky note or index card. Keep this phrase handy as you plan healthy changes. Create your non-negotiable behaviors. Practice reframing your thoughts (i.e., *I don't sit down to watch TV before going on a walk, I don't buy snack or junk foods that only tempt me to eat poorly, I don't stay up after 10:00 pm as I need my wind-down time, I don't eat after dinner,* etc.). Draft a few thoughts here.

   _____

   _____

   _____

   _____

3. Review the steps of the Healing Chronic Illness Overview. Which step needs the most attention to create your recovery story? Start there and craft your own plan. For true healing, reverse the brain patterns that keep you sick. Implement Build-A-Better-Brain healing practices multiple times per day. Do your best to see that you're spending at least an hour collectively each day on these practices. These are the building blocks of our recovery. Whether it's six blocks of 10 minutes, four blocks of 15 minutes, or two blocks of 30 minutes each, stack them throughout your day to rebuild a better brain. *Reclaim your physical and emotional health!*

_____

_____

_____

_____

SECTION NOTES:

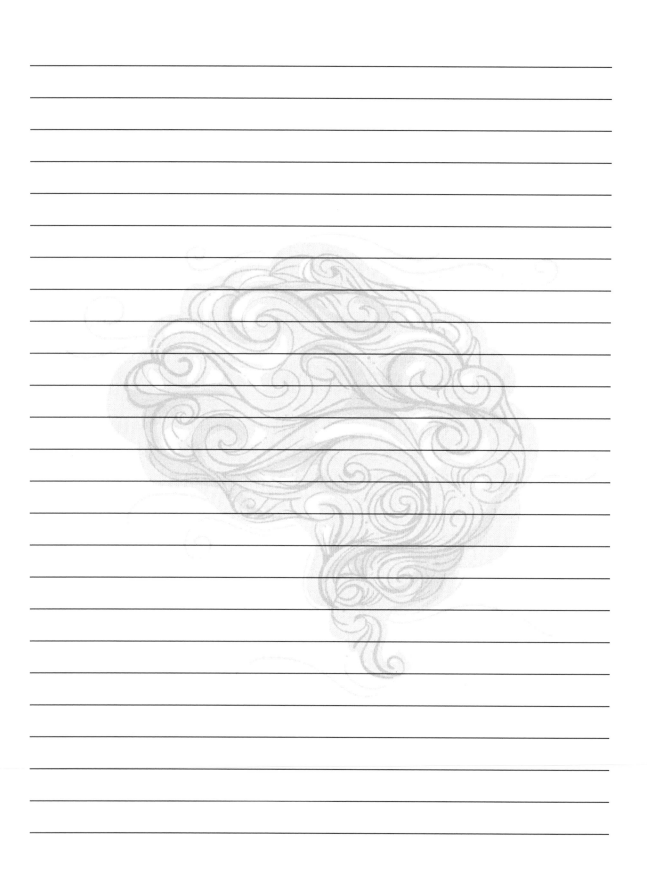

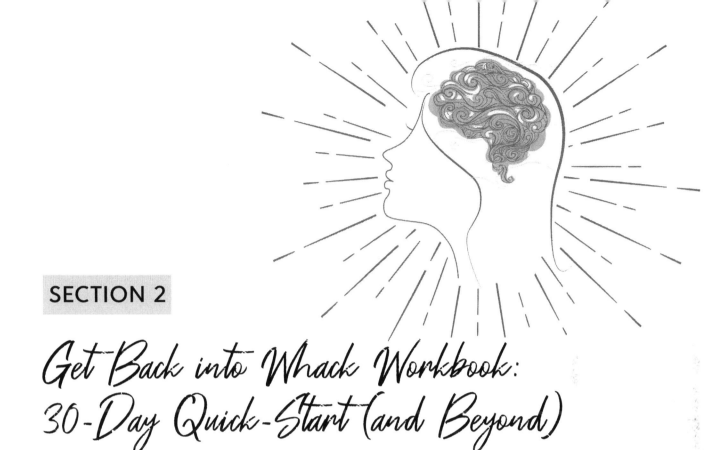

Get Back into Whack Workbook: 30-Day Quick-Start (and Beyond)

Welcome to the "Live It" section of this workbook. You've now answered and explored the Head Work questions from Section 1. You've taken action. The Head Work questions are designed to prompt changes in thinking patterns. Keep in mind that changing *how* you think *is* taking action.

Now, it's time to *Get Back into Whack!*

The following 30-Day Quick-Start section is divided into four main themes—each laying the foundation of a powerful core principle. Each theme offers a handful of practices to consider adding and engaging in daily. One topic builds upon the next.

This "one week at a time" pace allows you the freedom to focus on and gain mastery with one core principle before moving on. Don't skip ahead. This day-by-day process provides plenty of time to implement and tweak these activities. By strategically building your mental muscles in this way, you'll discover the satisfaction of weekly success and the motivation to continue moving forward. You'll embrace these core principles as your own.

> ***Upgrade your mind and body***
> ***to create the life and the future of your dreams.***

Choose a day to begin and jump in. Don't wait. There's no need to start on the first day of the year, month, or even week. Start NOW.

Week 1 – Upgrade with Gratitude

The theme for this week is gratitude, thankfulness, and appreciation. I've strategically chosen these words for the healing emotions they elicit. I can't overstate the importance here. These words evoke an emotional and physical response. This response—when amplified—serves as a natural autonomic nervous system (ANS) reset. It's part of the body's relaxation response.

Our daily stressors of dealing with life, work, relationships, and worries over our health add up. A chronically engaged stress response leads to deterioration of both the body and the brain.

The antidote? The relaxation response! An engaged relaxation response allows for:

- Hormonal balance and regulation
- An expanded sense of peace and calm
- Restored mental clarity
- Body system regulation that fosters whole-body healing
- And, much, much more

The practices shared this week offer fast and efficient methods to generate the very emotions and feelings we desire. Thankfully, they're also easy to do.

■ Practice #1.1 Gratitude Journal

The science is clear. Regular gratitude practices can lead to a greater sense of happiness, as well as other health benefits.[6] Feelings of gratitude help to reduce the effects of stress on the body. One simple and easy way to practice gratitude is to keep a journal. Jotting down things for which you're grateful shifts your focus in a positive direction. It encourages you to reflect upon your day in a rosy light, looking for the bright spots.

For a win/win experience, write in your gratitude journal at bedtime. Doing so shifts your focus away from the stress of the day and produces calming thoughts and feelings which prepare you for better sleep. This practice pairs perfectly with prayer and meditation.

---

6   https://www.health.harvard.edu/healthbeat/giving-thanks-can-make-you-happier

Don't overcomplicate things. Before bed tonight, grab a journal, notebook, or a plain pad of paper. Write down three things for which you're grateful. Make sure that you write down three *different* things each time that you practice this simple activity.

Make this a weekly practice. Write in your gratitude journal once per week[7] on the same day. Decide now which day you'll keep your gratitude practice. Regardless of what day you've chosen, **start tonight**. Then, do it again on the day of the week you've specified. For example, if today happens to be Tuesday, and you've decided to write in your gratitude journal on Sunday nights, go ahead and begin today. Then do it again on this coming Sunday (and Sundays thereafter).

I've taught this subject in workshops as well as frequently writing articles about it. (See "gratitude" in the Resources Guide in this workbook.)

■ Practice #1.2 Focus on Fulfillment

This fulfillment practice is a separate writing activity from your gratitude practice. It's your choice whether you use the same journal or notebook or something different.

Each evening, answer this question: *What did I accomplish today?*

Again, don't overcomplicate this. While most people ruminate at the end of the day on what didn't get done and what's left to do — that won't be you! Once you jot down your accomplishments for the day, you'll feel like a superstar.

The goal here is to make it quick. List the highlights of your day; no judgments allowed. List the tasks you completed — laundry, work reports, ferrying children, cooking or shopping, taking a walk, sorting through papers, meditating, paying bills, weeding, holding your tongue, deciding which cable service to use, etc. Whatever! Big or small, jot it down.

The purpose of this exercise is, again, twofold. This activity switches your focus toward something positive and productive, *and* it serves as a valuable future resource. On days where you feel that you're getting nowhere or feeling frustrated with yourself, flip back through your notes, and meditate on your accomplishments. This is a FEEL GOOD, "pat yourself on the back" activity.

---

7   https://nuvanna.com/the-gratitude-experiment/

> ***Remind yourself DAILY that you've
> done enough, and you ARE enough.***

Don't get sidetracked here. Only focus on the fulfillment side of things. And, let me clarify this next point. What you do in life does not determine your value. Even if you sit on the couch all day and feel that you achieve nothing, this exercise is **not** a reflection of your value or worth. This exercise is about recognition of who you are. If you spoke on the phone to anyone, were you kind? Take the time to look for what you accomplish each day. These reminders are powerful, and over time, they generate a deep sense of fulfillment. Moving toward a positive frame of mind is a choice. The more often you *choose* to do so, the easier it becomes.

Here's a Tony Robbins quote from a morning talk show discussion on priming the mind with meditation.

> ***"With our thoughts, we're either building
> a highway or a dirt road toward what we want.
> A highway is built with repetition;
> a dirt road with occasional use."***

This defines the benefit of neuroplasticity[8] (discussed more in *Get Back into Whack)*. We "build a highway" with the thoughts we think most often. The design of these exercises ensures that we employ the most constructive self-talk possible. I often think of this highway or dirt road analogy as I adopt intentional mindset or meditative practices. I hope you do too.

■ Practice #1.3 Sleep Hygiene

In addition to gratitude and a sense of fulfillment, sleep is a perfect way to restore homeostasis (maintaining a stable and constant level of health). Sleep is sometimes referred to as "the athlete's steroid"[9] because of its known performance-enhancing effects.

---

8   https://positivepsychology.com/neuroplasticity/
9   https://www.ideafit.com/fitness-library/sleep-the-athletersquos-steroid

Create your own sleep hygiene practice to ensure consistent and restorative levels of sleep. Review Callie's sleep hygiene example provided in Chapter 11 of *Get Back into Whack*. Before establishing practices that can help you to unwind, consider what pre-bedtime activities pose a challenge. What's in the way of better sleep for you?

- Inconsistent bedtimes and bedtime procrastination
- Before bed screen time[10] (electronics—TV, phone, tablet, computer, etc.)
- Distracting lights and noises in your bedroom
- Room temperature issues (too hot or too cold)
- Feelings of anxiety, worry, or restlessness that prohibit/prevent falling asleep
- Eating late—trying to sleep on a full stomach (or after eating unhealthy snacks)
- Interruptions from others—sounds or movements from a spouse, children, pets, etc.
- Sleep disrupting stimulants/depressants such as caffeine, alcohol, nicotine, sugar, etc.

Sketch out the basics of Callie's routine and adjust to make it your own. Brainstorm a list of activities that feel soothing to you. Consider restful activities such as reading, stretching, soft music, a bath/shower, restorative yoga, and aromatherapy with therapeutic essential oils. After your writing practice(s), prepare for sleep using prayer/meditation, deep breathing, self-hypnosis,[11] or guided imagery.

Create your practice with strategies tailored to you. A hot bath, for example, may sound blissful to one person and not-so for another. Make your sleep hygiene routine unique.

Write it, practice it, tweak it.

> ### *Healing begins with my thoughts.*

---

10   https://www.sleepfoundation.org/articles/why-electronics-may-stimulate-you-bed
11   https://mikemandelhypnosis.com/2018/02/23/self-hypnosis-easy-way/

Week 2 – Upgrade with Brain Retraining

The practices found in Week 1 (gratitude, fulfillment, and sleep) calibrate the body for healing and repair. This week amplifies these foundational principles.

Chapter 16 of *Get Back into Whack*, lists dozens of Build-a-Better-Brain practices. For the sake of simplicity, we'll focus on three in this section. You may wish to think of these as "before practices." It's handy to create a routine by doing these activities before something you do daily, such as before bed, work, or meals.

■ Practice #2.1 Top Off Your Inspiration Tank

Equip your mind with words, visuals, music, and images that keep you in a resourceful state. As a suggestion, begin your day with Positive Prime[12] sessions scientifically designed to improve mood, encourage self-acceptance, and generate feelings of contentment and happiness (https://www. positiveprime.com/). (*If you haven't set up your free account yet, use this link. And, if you'd be so kind, please enter my referral code,* **sue-1136***. Noting my referral code allows me to earn points to apply toward more Positive Prime sessions.*)

For optimal potential, here's how I apply these practices to my day. I do Positive Prime sessions before starting work in the morning and before getting back to it after lunch. I listen to relaxation sounds or ASMR[13] videos while I write and take frequent stretching breaks throughout the day (when I remember to set a timer). I also read Bible verses and devotionals.

To amp up my results, I often Tap[14] while I do positivity practices. If you're not Tapping regularly (I do it daily), you're missing out. Tapping is proven to lower stress hormones, such as cortisol.[15] And since stress gets in the way of a positive mindset, why not maximize your results? (See "tapping" in the Resources Guide of this workbook.)

Of course, use whatever brain-building practice(s) you prefer. Read, write, or doodle motivational quotes. Say mantras, affirmations, or afformations.® Journal, pray, and reflect on matters that help you to feel spiritually connected. Do a yoga pose. Take a walk in nature. Do whatever allows your body and brain opportunity to reset and recharge. At least four times per day, try to do a 15-minute

---

12   https://www.positiveprime.com/
13   https://www.youtube.com/watch?v=DxjfyBEIl7Q
14   https://rebuildingwellness.com/tapping-fibromyalgia/
15   https://www.thetappingsolution.com/blog/measurable-tapping-reduces-bodys-stress-hormones/

positivity practice. Or break it into two sessions of 30 minutes or even six sessions of 10 minutes each. Whatever works for you.

These practices are known to help stimulate the vagus nerve resulting in the body's calming response. Repeated practice is akin to finding the shut-off switch to the sympathetic nervous system/stress response.[16]

Desirable heart rate variability or HRV[17] (a helpful indicator of healthy vagal tone), is also achieved through these practices. Dr. Bessel van der Kolk has this to say about the importance of HRV, "We can actually change the state of our brain by what we do with our bodies. The way we move, the way we breathe, the way we interact with other people physically. HRV is a very important factor for the entire regulation of the complete system."[18]

These practices naturally improve and invite the state of coherence.[19]

Here's how Dr. Rollin McCraty, Research Director for the HeartMath Institute, defines it: "Coherence is the state when the heart, mind, and emotions are in energetic alignment and cooperation. It's a state that builds resiliency—personal energy is accumulated, not wasted—leaving more energy to manifest intentions and harmonious outcomes."

Select which practice(s) you *decide* to implement daily. View your practice as a non-negotiable; make it a consistent daily habit. Resist the temptation to skimp or skip, by focusing on the benefits of how you feel when you do them.

■ Practice #2.2 Deep Breathing Reset

Simple deep breathing exercises can be the fastest way to restore a sense of balance (and calm) to the body. Review the basic deep breathing examples in Chapter 9 of *Get Back into Whack*. Stressful circumstances throughout the day provide multiple opportunities to employ deep breathing techniques.

When you feel yourself taking short, shallow breaths—take one deep breath. Inhale through the nose and exhale slowly through the mouth (through pursed lips). Make the exhale slightly longer than the inhale. This fundamental reset may be all that you need.

---

16   https://www.thecut.com/2019/05/i-now-suspect-the-vagus-nerve-is-the-key-to-well-being.html
17   https://rebuildingwellness.com/hrv-fibromyalgia/
18   https://holisticchildpsychiatrist.wordpress.com/
19   https://www.heartmath.org/articles-of-the-heart/the-math-of-heartmath/coherence/

Additionally, consider making a deep breathing practice part of your routine as an hourly reset. Do you feel like that's too much to remember during your busy day? Here's a simple memory trick. Choose an arbitrary number between 1 and 60—the number 14, for example. Then take a deep breath (or several) at 14 minutes past each hour. You could also set a timer or write notes to yourself. The fact is, even if you follow through only 50% of the time, this results in doing deep breathing more than you do now. Your relaxed body is the beneficiary.

Have you downloaded the Pain Pathways app? (See "deep breathing" in the Resources Guide in this workbook.) Take advantage of the many guided audios—including deep breathing practices—that this helpful app has to offer.

■ Practice #2.3 Hydration Success

Do you experience any of these symptoms?

- Dry skin and/or dry eye
- Morning nausea
- Dark yellow/orange urine
- Constipation
- Impaired digestion, IBS, intestinal cramping
- Chronic coughs, sneezing, throat clearing, phlegm, sinus congestion
- Balance issues including weakness, dizziness, and instability
- Back pain
- Joint pain
- Muscle pain and spasms
- Increased and/or fluctuating heart rate
- Chills, fever, and body temperature fluctuation

These can all be symptoms of dehydration. Proper hydration is an essential part of staying healthy. It can aid in digestion, regulate body temperature, improve your body's ability to detoxify, and even decrease joint, back, and muscle pain.

When it comes to water, here's how the body stacks up. Our brain and heart are composed of 73%, lungs 83%, skin 64%, muscles and kidneys 79%, and our bones are made up of 31% water.[20]

---

20   https://www.usgs.gov/special-topic/water-science-school/science/water-you-water-and-human-body?qt-science_center_objects=0#qt-science_center_objects

Water is a fundamental nutrient.

If you currently don't drink much water, yet you don't feel thirsty, consider it a warning. Feelings of hunger are often masquerading for what is genuinely thirst. If you're hungry between meals, sip, sip, sip, rather than snack. The body requires sufficient quantities of pure, clean, filtered water for proper metabolism, nutrient absorption, and systemic regulation.

I shouldn't have to say this, but I will anyway. Please avoid sodas, sweetened blended drinks, sugary fruit smoothies, sports drinks, fruit juices (even 100% juice if processed), etc. Avoid caffeine and fake sweetened beverages, too. Also, avoid unfiltered tap water as it may contain harmful heavy metals and contaminants.[21]

Want more info on how much water to drink and when to drink? Download my handy—and free—water hydration tip sheet. (See "hydration" in the Resources Guide in this workbook.)

---

21   https://www.businessinsider.com/signs-tap-water-contaminated-unsafe-2019-5#other-contaminants-are-invisible-9

Week 3 – Upgrade with Body Mechanics

Most of us rarely consider the physical mechanics of how we move throughout our day. We assume that our bodies will comply with our desire to sit on the couch, stand in the kitchen, or walk to the mailbox. Some make fewer assumptions, others more.

Our bodies also assume. They assume the positions we practice the most. Over time our bodies "learn" how to slump, crouch, and constrict in harmful ways. To counteract this unnatural progression, we must become aware of how we use our physical structure—often referred to as body mechanics.

If you've ever worked out with personal trainers at the gym, they likely gave you a few pointers on body mechanics. They probably shared how to lift weights safely, and position your spine and legs to support you during your workout. The use of proper body mechanics isn't just for the gym. It's universally needed wherever you go. The topic of body mechanics includes posture, stamina, core strength, and coordination.

For this week, we'll concentrate mainly on posture.

Pay attention to your body. Do you sink into your chair or couch with your spine in a curved position? Do you hunch your neck forward as you type or look at your phone? Do you stand with your weight mainly on one leg with your knees locked?

This week's focus shares three basic practices. For more information on this powerfully healing subject, I recommend two books:

1. I've written an enthusiastic recommendation of Shoosh Lettick-Cotzer's book *Yoga for Fibromyalgia*. (See "yoga" in the Resources Guide in this workbook.)
2. I love the simple illustrations and do-able suggestions for a pain-free life from co-authors Lora Pavilack and Nikki Alstedter in their book, *Pain-Free Posture Handbook*.

I interviewed both Shoosh and Nikki while writing this workbook, and I share their juiciest tips on posture and body movement below.

■ Practice #3.1 Posture

Proper alignment of the body helps it work with efficiency. Yoga instructor and author Swoosh Lettick-Crotzer mentions that slouching compresses the torso, which compromises the rib cage and limits deep breathing. Poor posture restricts lymphatic flow, which we'll detail further in Week 4.

Yoga instructor and author Nikki Alstedter describes a favorite posture-enhancing position that's an easy way to "check-in" with your body. It can be done first thing in the morning, at night before bed, or both. This pose, called the Hook Lying Position,[22] is perfect for allowing the body to release tension in a safe and relaxed way.

To do: Lie flat on the floor or a mat with your knees bent and your feet hip-distance apart. Firmly ground your feet to the floor and relax your spine in a neutral position. Breathe deeply and allow the body to "settle" into relaxation and rest. You may wish to place the palms of your hands on the floor beside you, on your abdomen, or your heart. From this position, check-in with yourself. Plan the success of your day ahead or contemplate the achievements you've already had.

As you move throughout your day, consider your sitting posture. Nikki encourages us to think of our body like a snowman with three parts stacked on top of each other: the pelvis, chest, and head.

Consider how these parts stack in alignment as we sit. Nikki points out that the head weighs 7-10 pounds, and for every inch that it's thrust forward, it adds an extra load of 10 pounds onto the spine and the rest of the body.

Keep your head in alignment over your chest. Your ears should align with your shoulders. As an added tip, she suggests that we keep computer screens and electronics at eye level to minimize "tech neck" (a curved neck from consistently looking down at electronic devices).

Among many other useful illustrations, you can locate helpful diagrams of neck tension-releasing exercises on pages 98-99 of Nikki and Lora's book, *Pain-Free Posture Handbook.*

■ Practice #3.2 Physiology, Psychology, and Power Poses

If you haven't already, watch Amy Cuddy's TED talk on body language and Power Poses.[23] In it, she shares her insights into body language and how we can use it to our advantage. Her examples include job interviews and other corporate life scenarios.

---

22   https://www.verywellhealth.com/safely-release-your-back-muscles-with-hook-lying-296827
23   https://www.youtube.com/watch?v=Ks-_Mh1QhMc.

However, when you watch this useful talk, rather than focusing on the job interview aspect, think about how power poses and your posture relate to you. How do you stand, sit, or walk in everyday life? Your physiology has much to say. In particular, become aware of how your posture, stance, and body alignment affect your mood.

Yes, how you sit or stand affects how you feel.

Do you sit in a contracted position as if you're afraid to take up space in this world? Do you hold yourself in awkward poses or positions to "protect" yourself from pain or discomfort? Most of us are entirely unaware of how we present ourselves. It's a nonconscious behavior.

Whether you're in a group or all alone, notice what your body stance has to say. Notice how you feel. Positions of confidence (or power poses) can literally alter your brain chemistry.[24] So, why not put this helpful information to use?

If you're feeling sad, despondent, frustrated, isolated, etc. sit up (or stand) straight. Put a smile on your face (whether you think it's genuine or not), and straighten your shoulders back. Aligned posture can instantaneously invite feelings of empowerment, confidence, and motivation.

Find multiple pose options at TheRiseandShine.com.[25] Try them for yourself and modify as needed. Use whatever parts of these poses that make sense to you. Use them to boost your confidence and generate positive emotions.

Like most other positive practices that I do, I like to combine several. Strike a positive pose and repeat an affirmation, afformation®, or your favorite mantra. Sit up tall and Tap on whatever is bothering you at the moment. Use the resources you have to improve your mood at every turn.

Encourage your children and others to practice these simple adjustments, too. Remind them that their psychology affects their physiology and vice versa.[26]

> ***"Our bodies change our mind,***
> ***our mind changes our behaviors,***
> ***and our behaviors change our outcomes."***
> —Amy Cuddy

---

24   https://learningenglish.voanews.com/a/your-body-posture-can-change-your-brain/2710394.html
25   http://theriseandshine.com/4-ultimate-power-poses-help-feel-like-total-boss/
26   http://www.stress.org.uk/crucial-bear-mind-psychology-affects-physiology-vice-versa/

■ Practice #3.3 Universal Yoga Pose

When I asked Shoosh for a simple yoga pose that's easy to do, she was quick to respond. "One that I find to be most valuable for almost every person is called Viparita Karani or Legs Up the Wall.[27]* This pose is known for its stress relief benefits as well as helping with circulation in the legs. It also relaxes the muscles in the back, opens the chest, and encourages deeper breathing."

To do: Lie on the floor next to a couch, chair, or wall. Depending on your comfort level, raise your legs and rest them on a couch or chair seat, or directly up the wall. Use pillows, if needed, under the head, neck, sacral area, or wherever they may feel most comfortable. Optional—you may wish to listen to soothing music, employ aromatherapy, or practice your favorite breathing techniques while relaxing.

Breathe deeply and relax into this pose for 3-15 minutes, depending on your level of comfort.

As a regular practice, this pose offers a few moments for reflection and elicits a feeling of being centered as well as numerous physical benefits.

If you have a glaucoma diagnosis, discuss this and other yoga poses with your trusted medical professional before practicing.

---

27   https://www.yogajournal.com/poses/legs-up-the-wall-pose

Week 4 – Upgrade with Balance

This week is all about gaining balance in life. Becoming more aware of what we want in life sheds light on what's not working so well. Rather than dwell on the "not going so well," choose to focus on improvements that nudge momentum in the other direction.

Look for ways to balance your life in these critical areas: nutrition, stress management, relationships/ environment, and body movement. These areas reign supreme over your physical and emotional health.

■ Practice #4.1 Micro Goals

Choose a small goal you'd like to build into a healthy habit. Review those outlined in Chapter 6. For ease, I'll use a commonly chosen nutrition goal as an example.

Let's say the goal is to add more veggies to your diet. Consider several options for how to make it happen. You could browse a farmer's market, find a new, local produce store, or select an unfamiliar vegetable at a regular grocery store for a bit of variety. You could also take a cooking class, purchase an online meal plan, or buy cookbooks and magazines featuring recipes with a wide range of vegetables. There are dozens of ways to create micro-steps from any of these options.

One example of a micro-step is deciding to add a variety of greens to two out of three meals per day. You could include a salad or a serving of veggies to a meal. Even easier, consider serving whatever you're having on a bed of greens. Micro-steps are about simplicity.

For more information on why adding leafy greens can help you to heal from chronic illness, and how to make it a daily practice, check out my pertinent nutrition articles. (See "greens" in the Resources Guide in this workbook.)

Don't worry if your micro-step is so small that you feel you've nailed it in the first week. Continue to practice it for at least 30 days to solidify it as a habit. When one micro habit feels strong, add another. It's okay to add more than one micro-step at a time, but I'd suggest no more than three—and only if the steps are tiny.

Your micro-steps are unique to you. It's difficult to make general suggestions since readers have such diverse needs and starting places. You'll find a mini list of ideas below. Please adapt them to your own liking. If some are too simple, beef 'em up. If some are too challenging, ratchet 'em down a notch. The key is to tailor them to your own requirements.

Sample micro habits:

- Drink one glass of water ½ hour before meals (or less water if you currently drink very little)
- Practice Tapping (EFT) while stating your favorite prayer, meditation, affirmation, mantra, or afformation® while looking in the mirror after brushing your teeth
- March in place for five minutes before lunch (if you're mainly sedentary now)
- Roll your neck and/or shoulders three times per day after meals
- Eat one serving of berries with lunch on Mondays, Wednesdays, and Fridays
- Practice deep breathing each time you wash your hands
- Practice future pacing (designing your desired future) each morning as you wake and each evening before you fall asleep
- Repeat three of your favorite affirmations, mantras, or afformations® as you towel off after a bath or shower
- Dance, hop, jog or even wiggle to your favorite tunes before your workday begins

These are just a few ideas to prime your mental pump. What comes to mind for you?

■ Practice #4.2 Moving Meditations

Moving meditation activities provide a powerful way to incorporate both mind and body healing. Intentional and practiced movement can calm the brain, regulate breathing, ease digestion, improve overall systemic function, and reset hormonal regulation.

Healing body movement practices such as tai chi, qigong, and yoga are widely known for these benefits. Other activities can help, too. Walking, hiking, or biking in nature can enliven the senses and restore feelings of peace and calm. Swimming (especially in the ocean, rivers, or lakes) can also soothe the soul.

Range of motion activities—gentle stretching, walking, bouncing on a rebounder (mini-trampoline), aqua therapies, tai chi, yoga, qigong, etc.—can help to tone the body in ways that don't harm the joints. It takes time and nuanced practice to protect your boundaries of motion while continuing to challenge yourself (gently) to do more.

Shoosh encourages moving meditations—especially yoga—as there's much more going on than meets the eye. She says, "Slow, deep exhalations help to move the lymphatics. And because they regulate the immune system—there are even lymphatic vessels found in the brain—there's greater evidence of a connection between deep breathing practices and improvements in autoimmune conditions. Yoga, in particular, helps to expand the lungs and increase their capacity. Deep breathing while practicing slow, meditative exercises such as yoga draws more oxygen into the body. Expansion and contraction of the ribs also help to pump lymphatics through the body."

Shoosh summarizes her point with this statement, "Everyone can benefit by slowing down, resting, breathing deeply, and exercising." (See "moving meditations" in the Resources Guide in this workbook.)

■ Practice #4.3 The Cost of Clutter

Clutter causes sensory overload,[28] among other detrimental effects. It's known to add to the emotions of anxiety, stress, and feelings of overwhelm. I can attest to this first-hand, and maybe you can too. Some areas of my home stay neat and organized. Some do not. My office is a hodgepodge of tidy and serene vignettes, and areas that should be cordoned off with crime scene tape.

So, here goes. I'm practicing the following de-cluttering steps while I write so you won't feel alone.

1. **Choose** one area to begin (I'm choosing my desk's surface). Start small! One area—one drawer, one bookshelf, etc. Depending on the size, use large boxes or baskets for containment. (Laundry baskets make handy and efficient sorting bins.)
2. **Remove** everything from the area you wish to declutter. (Skipping this step doesn't work. If you try to merely thin the clutter, you're left with the same one-at-a-time decision-making issues that caused the problem in the first place.)
3. Once it's cleared, **sort** through the objects (quickly) for what stays and what goes (donate or toss). Consider in advance the overall look you want to achieve. Then assess the items accordingly, comparing them to see if they "fit" into your desired mental scheme.
4. **Clean** the area that's now cleared of clutter—vacuum, mop, dust, scrub, or polish as needed.
5. **Replace** items you've decided to keep. Arrange them according to your pre-planned notion of how you want that area to look and feel.
6. **Toss** your discard pile into the trash. Take your **donate** box directly to a thrift store or reclamation center. Or, put the box in your car and commit to a drop off date.
7. **Enjoy** and admire your work. Pat yourself on the back for a task well done.

My desk looks great! I hope your decluttering project goes well, too. With this sense of accomplishment in place, plan and schedule the next area you wish to tackle.

---

28   https://www.fastcompany.com/3052894/7-ways-clutter-is-ruining-your-life

*"When we clear the physical clutter from our lives,
we literally make way for inspiration
and 'good, orderly direction' to enter."*
—Julia Cameron

SECTION NOTES:

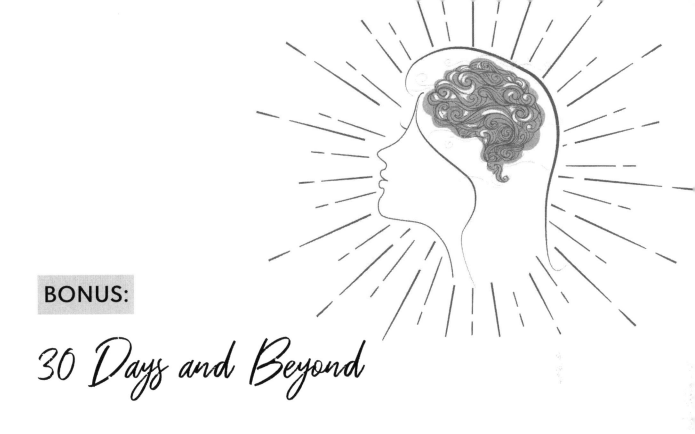

30 Days and Beyond

Welcome to your **Weekly Theme Action Guide**!

Now that you've built a strong foundation over the past month, it's time to flex those mental muscles and add more practices to bolster what you've learned.

Below, you'll find themes to add to your *Get Back into Whack* plan for an additional eight weeks. This workbook can take you a full 90 days and beyond.

There's flexibility here. Either follow the weekly schedule as listed or use your intuition to guide you to the theme to implement next (I recommend implementing weeks 11 and 12 last). Whether you apply the remaining eight themes in numerical order or your desired sequence, I suggest you write them out on a calendar for easy viewing. **The order of the following subjects may not be vital, but each one is**. Meaning, refrain from cherry-picking some themes and omitting others. It's essential to implement them all.

Week 5 – Theme: POWER WORDS

Do you remember this characteristic of the nonconscious mind as outlined in Chapter 2 of *Get Back into Whack?*

- The **nonconscious mind** is highly symbolic and thinks in terms of pictures, words, images, sounds, and feelings.

What does highly symbolic mean? The nonconscious mind makes mental pictures of images, symbols, words, animals, objects, or people. It also adds emotions and feelings to these representations.

Abstract subjects such as time or strategic plans are not part of nonconscious programming. Putting this knowledge to use, we can use symbols—especially words—to plant the seeds of our desired future.

Here are a few ways we can use words to fuel our plans for growth:

- Positive coloring and activity books such as *Chronic Coloring* (find on Amazon)
- Word clouds[29]
- Vision boards[30]
- Quote books
- Bible verses and devotionals
- Affirmations, afformations®, mantras*
- Card decks and flashcards
- Audios of positive statements (pre-recorded)
- Audios of positive statements (record your own)
- Music with positive and uplifting lyrics

*Quick definitions of these often-recommended positivity practices:

Affirmations—Positive statements that express what you'd like to create more of in your life. They reflect the actions, desires, or circumstances that you'd like to come to fruition.

---

29   https://www.wordclouds.com/
30   https://rebuildingwellness.com/positive-future/

Afformations®—"Empowering questions that immediately change your subconscious thought patterns from negative to positive," says originator Noah St. John.[31] (Please review the citation below for more information on how to form these provocative yet simple questions.)

Mantras—Positive phrases or statements repeated for emphasis. My favorite way to use mantras comes from the work of Dana Wilde of *Train Your Brain* fame and the Mind Aware Show.[32] She recites positive statements about her goals and creates them on the spot. The spontaneity, along with emphasis, creates motivation and anticipation of success. As she gets going and amps up her excitement for what she wants, she sometimes calls her mantras, rants.[33] Whether you're reciting a positive mantra or ranting about the positive things you can see happening around you, it's all good. They're both great ways to generate positive emotions.

Use positive words to your advantage!

Write positive statements on index cards, sticky notes, journals, or notes on your phone. Use lipstick or dry-erase markers to write on your mirrors. To help you reframe and reshape your thoughts, write positive words and phrases wherever you'll see them most. Practice your favorite methods of positivity statements and repeat them often. Say them aloud. Tap, walk, or exercise as you recite them.

With intention, decide to choose empowering, helpful, and supportive inner language. For more information on the definitions and differences between affirmations, afformations,® and mantras, check out my articles on the subject and others. (See "healing words" in the Resources Guide in this workbook.)

Bonus tip: Fill the Void.

Get Back into Whack contains numerous references to thought patterns related to our MAPP. The frequent use of the word "pattern" is intentional for the mental representation it creates. A pattern defines the outline or the guideline to what's expected.

Paper sewing patterns, for example, are specifically designed to make one unique item. It's a sure thing. Pattern pieces designed to create a skirt provide precise cutting guides, and after sewing the fabric pieces together, you have—voila!—a skirt. No surprise. There's no worry that we'll end up with a pair of jeans, is there?

---

31 https://noahstjohn.com/positive-affirmations-and-afformations-regular/
32 https://danawilde.com/show/
33 http://www.danawilde.com/HowToRant

Our mental patterns work in the same way. Our thoughts create predictable results. Noticing what they are can help us to forecast our outcomes with reliability.

We all have "fall back" thought patterns — thoughts that our mind habitually goes to. Our fall back patterns become most apparent in unguarded moments where our mind wanders. This can happen when showering, brushing teeth, or sitting at a traffic light.

Once we've decided to change our thinking patterns, it's not as simple as plucking out the negative ones. The mind doesn't like a vacuum. It will tend to go back to the same way of thinking, filling in new (yet similar) thoughts from our familiar internal repertoire. However, we can use this natural tendency to our advantage. We can replace what we remove with new thoughts — better thoughts.

> ### Choose *your thought patterns.*
> ### *Don't allow them to run on default.*

Keep it simple. Write a favorite quote or affirmation on an index card or your phone. Choose one quote. Refer to and repeat it each time you find yourself slipping into old familiar thought patterns. Repeat this "new and improved" thought until it's ingrained enough to pop into your head automatically.

Here are a few affirmation options to sample:

- I am whole, and I am healing.
- I nourish my body every day with healthy, whole, natural foods.
- I strengthen my body with daily fitness activities.
- I enjoy and crave nutrient-dense, fiber-rich foods.
- I'm thankful for my body. It's getting stronger and healthier every day.
- I'm so grateful that I grow in confidence daily.
- I enjoy a life filled with people, circumstances, and experiences I love.
- I succeed with grace, ease, and consistency.
- I practice what I want in life.
- My body is my house, and I choose to take care of it.
- I'm grateful for how my body supports me.

Jot down ideas of your own. Don't worry about getting it "right." Instead, use your intuition to write down what feels important and validating to you. You may also wish to seek out samples of affirmations, afformations®, or mantras to give you more guidance.

_____

_____

_____

_____

_____

_____

_____

> **"Worry is like a rocking chair. It gives you something to do, but it won't get you anywhere."**
> —Glenn Turner

I often work with private clients to help them create their own affirmations, mantras, and afformations®. If you'd like guidance in this area, contact me here: https://rebuildingwellness.com/contact/.

Week 6 – Theme: RESILIENCE

Resilience is a trending and popular topic in the self-development world. Along with grit and leaning in, resilience is a crucial characteristic often attributed to those who have overcome significant odds. I think of it as the ability to pick yourself up by your bootstraps and bounce back.

My wish is for you to build long-term resilience. I want you to not only bounce back from life's daily tussles but also from ones that are ongoing and may feel insurmountable.

Here are two fundamental principles that can lead to a life of resilience. Practice these daily and notice a positive shift in your viewpoint of relationships and interactions.

1. **The Casual Observer**. (Mentioned in Chapters 16 and 18 of *Get Back into Whack*.)

    This principle is about viewing a circumstance in retrospect (or in real-time) without judgment. Do this by playing the mental movie of the event through the lens of a third, uninvolved party. For example, imagine a disagreement between yourself and your boss. Imagine that you left his or her office feeling angry, unheard, and frustrated. Use the casual observer method to re-visit the scene. This time, in your mind's eye, see it unfold as if you're watching from a distance. Imagine viewing everything through the lens of a camera mounted in an upper corner of the room.

    From this vantage point, notice the happenings of the meeting. Replay the meeting in your mind. Use this non-judgmental viewpoint and observe the body language of both parties. Notice movements and facial expressions. Pay attention to not only what's said, but *how* it's said. Notice the posture and gestures of both parties as the conversation ends. Did you notice anything different or surprising from this perspective? Anything new?

    The casual observer perspective allows you to gain insight. As an added benefit, it promotes the ability to distance yourself from emotionally charged events. From this angle, you may be able to objectively remove yourself (or others) from blame, guilt, expectations, and more.

2. **Apply Self-Compassion**.

    Self-compassion may be a natural outcropping of principle #1. When you're able to view circumstances with an unattached viewpoint (a casual observer), it's more likely that you can recognize (and feel) the need for self-compassion.

One universal characteristic I uncover with chronic illness clients, is their relentlessly harsh and critical self-talk. Criticisms, reproaches, and accusations never generate positive behavior. Treating yourself with kindness is the first step toward building a better relationship with both your body and the world around you.

Apply self-compassion to your own thoughts and actions. When you judge yourself, you judge others too. In doing so, you effectively hand your power over to them. This power shift is a result of the "I'll be happy when" scenario. You've placed your sense of happiness in someone else's hands.

I encourage you to take it back.

Allow happiness into your life! Invite it through kindness and self-compassion. Use the casual observer viewpoint to revisit situations or to view them in real-time. Apply these simple practices and become resilient.

TIP: *Resilience can strengthen by all the brain-healthy practices mentioned in this workbook. Methods that calm and relax the autonomic nervous system (ANS) in general and the vagus nerve specifically, can help us to feel centered and whole. The vagus nerve is known for its multi-systemic connections, so restoring vagal tone creates body-wide healing benefits. One simple way is to relax the facial muscles and, in particular, the jaw. (We tend to clench our teeth and jaw when stressed). Allow the jaw to drop open just a bit and hum.*

Humming washes the body in a soothing, healing vibration. Hum whatever feels right to you. It could be a familiar melody, a single tone (such as saying "om"), or a specific humming technique such as the humming bee meditation.[34]

---

34   http://thehealthylivinglounge.com/2009/08/06/12-instant-benefits-of-humming-daily/

Week 7 – Theme: VALUES

This week, it's time to focus on what's important to you in life. We'll take a look at your priorities and interests by assessing your values.

What activities do you participate in most? Do your actions reflect what you want to do or what you believe you have to do?

Of course, life isn't all about doing what we want whenever we want. However, we must strike a balance between our have-to-do's and our want-to-do's.

It's very important to assess where these imbalances may lie, because they're often hidden or masked. To get to the heart of this challenge, answer the following survey questions with as much detail as possible:

1. *Other than work (if applicable), what do you do with most of your time?*

_____

_____

2. *What area of your life do you feel the most confident about? Where are you reliable, dependable, and disciplined?*

_____

_____

3. *In life's quiet moments, what do you dream of?*

_____

_____

4. *What inspires you?*

_____

_____

5. *What's your favorite topic or activity to explore and learn more about?*

_____

_____

6.   *What's most important to you about your health? (Write out at least 6-10 responses.)*

_____

_____

_____

_____

_____

_____

7.   *What's most important to you about your financial security? (Write out at least 6-10 responses.)*

_____

_____

_____

_____

_____

_____

8.   *What's most important to you about your spiritual life? (Write out at least 6-10 responses.)*

_____

_____

_____

_____

_____

9.   *What's most important to you about your creative life? (Write out at least 6-10 responses.)*

_____

_____

_____

_____

_____

_____

10.   *What's most important to you about your physical body, i.e, your appearance, strength, energy levels, etc.?*
       (Write out at least 6-10 responses.)

_____

_____

_____

_____

_____

_____

11.   *What's most important to you about your relationships? (Write out at least 6-10 responses.)*

_____

_____

_____

_____

_____

_____

12.   *What's most important to you about your sense of altruism, charity, or being of service? (Write out at least*
       6-10 responses.)

_____

_____

_____

_____

_____

_____

13. *In what area(s) — specifically — do you spend most of your money? (Not including housing and/or auto expenses.)*

_____

_____

14. *Do you have better success following through with your goals and plans under the support and guidance of someone else? Who would be a good accountability partner, coach, or mentor for you?*

_____

_____

15. *Review the above answers and write a comprehensive list of values that you feel are most important.*

_____

_____

_____

_____

_____

_____

For ideas and guidance on this topic, use my downloadable Core Values Checklist. (See "values" in the Resources Guide in this workbook.)

After compiling your list of values, list your top 10 below. Write them in order of importance and then highlight the top three.

_____

_____

_____

_____

There you have it — your personalized list of values!

This list can serve you in unexpected ways. In addition to helping align your goals, refer to your values list when looking for business or relationship partners. Use this list as you apply for new jobs or consider career changes. Use it as you make other life changes, too, such as moving to a new neighborhood, city, or state.

For now, let's crystallize your goals with the information you've gleaned from this work. Take your values list and review your goals as outlined in Chapter 6 of *Get Back into Whack* (or in this workbook). Notice how your goals align (or perhaps don't align) with your values.

Rewrite, tweak, add to, and adjust your goals as needed.

Here's an illustration of tweaking a health goal. Let's say that you wish to create a consistent deep breathing practice. After completing your values assessment, you note that financial security is a primary value for you, and you happen to sometimes fall into the trap of impulse spending. You could add to your goals list a suggested practice of taking three deep meditative breaths before making any purchase over a specific dollar amount. This alignment takes advantage of a skill you already want to improve (remembering to do deep breathing) and adding it to a circumstance that supports your values.

Applying your values to your goals list helps to bring a sense of clarity to what you want to achieve. ***Alignment between values and goals strengthens them both***.

Be sure to make multiple copies of both your values list and your current goals. Keep them handy and refer to them often. Notice how clarifying your values brings your choices into focus. Your values list can make most decision-making processes more straightforward.

Week 8 – Theme: SELF-CARE

This week's focus is all about YOU.

How well do you take care of yourself? *Where* are you on your to-do list for the day? Is the care and feeding of you a priority in your life?

These may sound like simple questions, but they're not. If you haven't noticed yet, many of us (okay, all of us) tend to say one thing but do another when it comes to self-care. We may want to get outdoors for a walk and shred some kale for lunch, but that's not always how the day turns out. Life has a way of overwriting our best-laid plans.

I get it.

That's why this week's focus is on turning that circumstance around. Take the opportunity now to discover what you can do to improve your self-care skills. The key is to make it simple.

The following is the most dangerous response given when I suggest specific self-care practices: *I'll do that when I have time (or money, or obtain a particular resource, etc.).*

> ### *Self-care needs to be primary, not an afterthought.*

The definition of self-care is entirely personal. One may feel manicures, for example, are necessary and mandatory. Another may think of them as an occasional pampering event. Compile your self-care list and remember that it's for you alone. Re-order topics according to what's important to you. Start with the suggestions below and then add your own ideas keeping in mind that it's about practicing the following, not perfection.

Non-negotiable self-care basics:

Nutritious Meals * Meditation and Prayer * Restorative Sleep * Fitness/Body Movement Activities * Water/Hydration * Daily Positivity Statements * Regular Dental Care[35] * Socialization and Making Human Connections[36] * a Regular Practice of Community and Fellowship * Creative Activities *

---

35   https://rebuildingwellness.com/dental-fibromyalgia/
36   https://rebuildingwellness.com/isolation-fibro/

Skin/hair/nail Care * Walking[37] or Stretching * Spiritual Support and Soul Connections * Deep Breathing Practices * Family Fun * Connecting with Nature * Saying, "I Love You" * Hugs (giving and getting)

Additional self-care activities to consider:

Dry Skin Brushing[38] * Massage[39] * De-cluttering * Doting on Your Pet * Adopting a Pet * Fun Outings with Friends * Coloring or Activity Books * EFT/Tapping * Creative Arts * Listening to or Creating Music * Reading[40] * Far Infrared Saunas * Aromatherapy with Pure Essential Oils * Magnesium Bath Soaks[41] * Memorize and Repeat Favorite Bible Verses * Smile at a Stranger * Memorize and Repeat Favorite Positivity Statements or Quotes * Gratitude and Thankfulness Practices * Manicures and/or Pedicures * Travel * Laughter * Getting Your Hair Done * Solitaire and Mindless Games * Invite a Co-Worker, Neighbor, or Acquaintance Over for Dinner * Libraries, Museums, and/or Galleries * Parks, Beaches, Lakes, or Rivers * Board Games * Grounding (stand on the dirt or grass with bare feet) * Bike Riding * Picnicing * Gardening * Pay It Forward * Do a Handicraft * Self-Hypnosis * Enjoy a Porch or Park Swing * Ask for Help * Inspirational Quotes * Inspirational Documentaries * Watching Silly Cat/Dog Videos * Aqua Therapy * Vision Boards * Road Trips * Stretches, Yoga, Tai Chi, or Qigong * Weighted Blankets[42] * Calling Friends * Napping * Watching Movies * T-Tapp[43] * Host a No-Special-Reason Party * Reconnecting With Old Friends * Play * Local School Sporting Events * Journaling * Goofing Off and/or Playing with Children * Inspirational Podcasts * Learning Something New * Jigsaw Puzzles (my fav!) * Forgiving Someone * Volunteering * Donating (time, money, resources) * Reading or Watching Something Fun * Spending Some Time in the Sun * Foam Rollers[44] * Learning How to Practice Self-Care from Your Pet[45] * a Quick Get-Away or a Staycation * Watching a Sunrise/Sunset * Watching Clouds * Watching Classic Films * Reading a Joke Book * Visiting an Animal Shelter and Donating old Towels and Blankets *

These are just some of the high spots. What else is on your self-care list? What's important to you and feeds your soul? Add more thoughts below.

---

37   https://rebuildingwellness.com/walking-energy-clarity-stability/
38   https://rebuildingwellness.com/dry-skin-fibro/
39   https://rebuildingwellness.com/chronic-pain-relief/
40   https://simontownley.com/storytelling/story-simplified/people-read-for-the-endorphins-and-the-cortisol-and-for-emotional-exercise/
41   https://rebuildingwellness.com/chronic-magnesium/
42   https://rebuildingwellness.com/fibromyalgia-weighted-blanket/
43   https://www.t-tapp.com/
44   https://rebuildingwellness.com/pain-hotspots/
45   https://rebuildingwellness.com/teacher-have-fur/

_____

_____

Once you've reviewed the list, get out your calendar, and enter in the non-negotiables that aren't happening now. For example, designate a regular time for shopping or prepping healthier foods. Schedule daily meditation practices, etc. Circle the ideas that spark interest for you and add them to your calendar. ***Scheduled events get done.***

For more reasons to make self-care a priority, check out several articles I've written on the subject. (See "self-care" in the Resources Guide in this workbook.)

Week 9 – Theme: MEASURED SUCCESS

I want you to be as successful as humanly possible. I'm sure you want that too.

This week's focus is all about tracking so that you can fortify your chances of success using scientifically proven methods. You're more likely to stay on track when progress is reviewed and recorded. Studies reveal, "Frequent monitoring of progress toward goals increases the chance of success."[46]

Keep this process simple. Rather than creating complicated multi-page spreadsheets or posters which can make the task feel like a drudge, I use a standard blank calendar. Whether digital or paper, create a system of monitoring that works best for you. Add an asterisk, for example, on the days that you've practiced meditation of some sort. Add an X or check mark on days you've exercised. Do whatever it is that makes progress visually recognizable.

Tracking on paper can create flexible options. You can print out a blank monthly calendar or use a pre-printed one. I like to use colored pens or highlighters so that at a glance, I can see how I'm doing. You may wish to use stickers or anything else that piques your interest.

For some projects or goals, I also use weekly or monthly checklists. These are useful to see your overall progress at-a-glance. Lists have another added benefit. They give you that "feel good" experience of marking things off as done. Don't discount this. A popular productivity site shares this fact, "Checking items off of a checklist releases small amounts of dopamine that then fuel us to keep checking off more items, i.e., get more done!"[47] The emotional benefit (aka the dopamine hit) contributes toward feelings of motivation as well as accomplishment.

To keep things interesting, make your tracking guides fun and eye-catching. Whether you use calendars, apps, spreadsheets, checklists, or to-do lists, make them your own by using (or choosing) your favorite methods, colors, and images.

Do you share your progress?

That's up to you. You get to choose whether to share your tracking guides with anyone else or not. For some, family and friends are supportive; for others, they're not. Of course, these tools are a perfect fit to share and support you within a mentorship or coaching relationship.

---

46   https://www.sciencedaily.com/releases/2015/10/151029101349.htm
47   https://blog.trello.com/the-psychology-of-checklists-why-setting-small-goals-motivates-us-to-accomplish-bigger-things

For additional information on Motivation and Tracking, check out the variety of articles I've written. (See "motivation" in the Resources Guide in this workbook.)

> ***"What's measured improves."***
> —Peter Drucker

Week 10 – Theme: (INTERNAL) PARTS DISCOVERY

In case you don't know it, inside your head is a complex mass of conflicting desires.

Yes, there may be many things you want to do, but if you're not viewing your motivation from this helpful perspective, you're hindered before you begin.

Does that surprise you?

Evaluating your internal parts is a powerful part of self-awareness. While it's probably unfamiliar, it provides a distinctive way to view how your desires, behaviors, and interactions with the world around you make sense to various aspects of yourself.

This week, your task is to focus on the parts of you that may not want to move forward. Do you feel a tug or even a dragging sensation when you think about starting a new routine? What about getting your feet out the door to walk, stretch, swim, or try a new fitness class? You may have a strong desire to build your body in healthy ways (I hope so!), but it's also likely that part of you is resistant.

That's okay.

Keep in mind that ***every single thought you have has a positive intention and deserves to be heard***. The one unifying goal for each of our internal parts is safety. If part of you wants to start an exercise program and part of you doesn't, something must feel unsafe or unsure to the resistant part.

Here's an excellent investigative question. Ask it in relation to a goal you've not yet achieved. "What am I afraid of giving up if I do X?" This prompt can help elicit the fears and objections the unsafe part of you believes to be true.

Fill in your answer below.

_____

_____

_____

_____

_____

Your thoughts and desires are reflections of the various parts of you. Not all are ready to shake their pom-poms at the notion of change. It's perfectly natural (and even primitively ingrained) to want to avoid change. It's your task then, to work *with* this natural tendency rather than against it.

The first step is to listen. Listen to the voice (the part of you) that wants to say no, the voice that wants to resist, discourage, and stop you from moving forward. This part is merely playing its role in trying to keep you safe. Listen to what it has to say without judgment or disapproval.

Pay attention to the objections that come forward. Address what you can and then redefine the purpose and reasons for your goal.

The second step is to move forward, anyway. While listening and understanding are essential, so is taking action even when things don't line up neatly. I'll say that again. In this instance, your ducks are not only *not* in a row; they're a scattered mess. That's okay. An aligned perspective is all that's needed as well as just one or two ducks in sight. Breaking the chain of stagnation is a powerful method to rewire the brain in ways that serve you today and for a lifetime.

There's a common adage in the neuroscience world referring to neuroplasticity that says, "Neurons that fire together wire together." Meaning, we build stronger pathways in areas of often-repeated thoughts and actions.

You're probably familiar with that phrase, but has the following occurred to you?

> ### *Breaking patterns can be equally as powerful as creating them.*

It's exciting to discover that neuroplasticity works in both directions. Repeated thoughts and behaviors build strengthened neural connections. And, when we *break undesired familiar patterns* (that have created robust neural connections), we weaken these pathways.

An example of unwanted eating patterns aptly demonstrates this point. Thoughts of loneliness, sadness, fear, anger, boredom, indecision, anxiety, etc. often prompt unhealthy mindless eating. Looping thoughts (those with no resolve) can trigger frustrating emotional eating behaviors.

By feeling a (perceived) negative emotion and then *not* eating something unhealthy, we can weaken the pattern and reduce its pull on us over time. (Spoiler Alert: This feels pretty cruddy at first. It's not a one-and-done fix. It takes time and repetition to break patterns just as it does to build them.)

TIP: *Neuro-Linguistic Programming (NLP), Tapping, and hypnosis practices can serve as powerful tools to help support and break undesirable patterns.*

I challenge you to play a game of "what if" this week. What if you have a thought that usually prompts a negative behavior—but you don't act on it? If a consistent exercise routine is on your wishlist, yet part of you wants to skip it because you're too tired, busy, or hungry, think about this: What if you felt those things, but you got in a quick workout anyway?

What if you felt annoyed by a co-worker's thoughtless comment, yet you *didn't* go to the breakroom for a donut? What if you built new healthy patterns based on what you *are* doing as much as what you aren't? It's certainly something to think about.

The more you practice breaking old behaviors and building new ones—by listening to all parts of you—the more centered and powerful you'll become.

> **"Depending on what they are, our habits will either make us or break us. We become what we repeatedly do."**
> —Sean Covey

Week 11 – Theme: A REARVIEW LOOK

You've come a long way. Seriously.

The challenge is how to make that fact seem tangible. How do you quantify it? It's human nature to feel we haven't made much progress no matter what we've done. We're programmed to put more focus on what we have yet to do or what we believe we've tried yet failed to do. That negative angle, while part of our instinctual response, is a sure-fire motivation buzzkill.

Instead, it's time to take a look at what you HAVE accomplished.

Let your past hard work serve you in the present. Locate the journal(s) you've been using since Week 1. Flip through the pages that list things for which you're grateful and review your entries containing the accomplishments you've made. Review the goals outlined in Section 1 of this workbook. Notice how you rated your desires, beliefs, and commitments. Now view them from today's perspective. How have these ratings changed?

Take a deep breath.

Settle into the present moment and feel the weight of the time and energy you've put into your goals over the past weeks or months. Study this workbook, your journals, calendars, and tracking notes. Fan through the pages. Read and re-read them. Notice your own handwriting and recall how you felt at the time of each entry. When you consider the invested time and energy, you'll recognize how far you've come.

Let this acknowledgment of time and progress resonate with your soul. That may sound a little airy-fairy, but I want you to allow this experience to reach more than your mind. I want you to *feel* it, too. I love the word resonate. To let something resonate means to allow it to create a sound or vibration within you. Musical tones harmonize and resonate with each other. And at an energetic level, emotions (especially gratitude, thankfulness, and appreciation) can create a vibrational resonance within us. We can feel an internal buzz.

Instead of focusing on the negative—a motivational buzzkill—focus on what you *have* accomplished. Create what I like to call a buzz-fill.

Once you feel that sense of resonance, then dig a little deeper. Review your progress and look for patterns. Do you notice any repeated stumbling blocks? What about times or areas of more considerable forward momentum? Use this vantage point to make discoveries about what holds you back and what gives you the juice to keep going. Add this new information to your already growing arsenal of skills. You know so much more now than you did when you first began. All of these learned behaviors fortify your motivation to continue.

For this week, engage in and immerse yourself in this buzzy feeling of satisfaction. Enlist and truly *feel* the resonance. Notice how this feeling energizes and feeds your soul. Also, notice the intentional choices of *what* you're reviewing. We naturally tend to look back at our lives and focus on our perceived failings. This week's theme offers an opposite approach. The skill of looking back at the positives provides you with the benefits acquired from focusing on what has gone *right*. You're looking back on the journey of where you were as opposed to where you are today.

Don't forget to reward* yourself as you go. Reflect on past accomplishments and give yourself recognition for your "in the moment" successes, too. Studies have shown that rewarding yourself in small ways right after completing micro tasks (immediacy is important) gives you a better overall feeling of accomplishment than waiting until later.[48]

I know I say this quite often, but please don't skip this step.

Small micro-steps in progress are proven to be most effective for long-term success. But it's a challenge to see micro progress. That's why this week's focus is so enlightening. Rather than going along with the status quo, build a future by looking back (through a constructive lens). This builds confidence, which leads to motivation. Continue to reward yourself and acknowledge your progress.

Post this on your bathroom mirror and repeat daily: **Little steps now, big results later. My progress is amazing!**

As a reminder, please don't use food or shopping as a reward. Anything that encourages unplanned eating and/or spending can burden your waistline or budget. For soul-supporting ideas on easy-to-implement rewards, check out this article featuring 50 ways to reward yourself without eating or spending money.[49]

---

48   https://www.biospace.com/article/new-research-suggests-frequent-rewards-can-improve-motivation-performance-at-work/
49   https://yesandyes.org/2015/10/rewards-that-arent-food-or-shopping.html

Week 12 – Theme: IDENTITY SHIFTS

I prefer to share some abstract topics, such as identity, in person rather than using an arm's length medium like writing. But here I go anyway. I'm diving in and promise to do my best.

When I work one-on-one with clients, I not only help them to make outward changes to their lives, I help them to make inward changes, too. These changes have the potential to serve them for a lifetime.

Here's a real-world example. Years ago, I worked with a young woman who had the typical college-age diet of pizzas, sodas, coffee drinks, crackers, chips, and breakfast cereals (for any meal of the day). She often grabbed her "meals" at convenience stores and drugstore checkout stands.

Her symptoms were apparent. She had skin rashes, acne, lack of energy, gut dysfunction, joint pain, and a family history of rheumatoid arthritis. Fearing what may be ahead for her, she contacted me, and we quickly got to work.

She was an extraordinarily bright and willing client. Together, we came up with healthier meal plans and ways to incorporate higher-quality foods into her busy life. She noticed symptom reductions right away. The first to go were the rashes and acne. I have to say she was more pleased with that than with just about anything else we did. Her body showed—by her symptoms—that it was not a fan of both processed dairy and the wheat/gluten found in manufactured food products. By weaning off these foods that contributed to her physical grief, she began to heal.

A few months after our start together, I taught a hands-on 12-week workshop on nutrition. She eagerly participated and helped me with some of the class materials and demonstrations. She also fielded questions from attendees about her own healing journey and experiences with me. I was tickled pink to hear the pride in her voice as she shared what she'd done to improve her quality of life.

I overheard someone tell her, "I couldn't live without cereal. I have it every day, and I don't know what I'd eat instead." My client's response surprised me. She said, "Oh, it's easy. I've never really liked cereal, but I enjoy filling up on veggies, salads, and other foods I make myself. They make me feel full and give me lots of energy. And my skin has never looked better!"

What was going on? I know she believed those things to be true now, but what about the past? Was she trying to hide her former food behaviors, or did she not remember how she used to eat?

Later, during one of our sessions, I casually asked her how she felt about bread, crackers, chips, and cereals. She said, "You know, I never really ate that much of them. I think I just knew that they made me sick."

That's when I discovered the powerful identity shifts that can happen from transformational healing work.

She no longer thought of herself as someone who ate with no regard of how it affected her. She made food choices as someone who respected her body and knew the consequences. She actually "forgot" her former self and became a new person with her new identity as a healthy eater. This phenomenon no longer surprises me as I see it happen over and over.

This week's focus is about understanding how you can alter your point of view paradigm. Adjusting how you view a particular topic can thereby change who you are at your core.

Core beliefs *can* change into new and improved beliefs.

One reason to create a values list (as detailed in Week 7), is to fortify our motivation by reviewing them. We can revisit this list periodically as we grow in our understanding of the lifestyle changes we wish to make. Over time, some values remain in the same position as before, while others may move up or down on the list. Also, we may have new ones to add and others to remove.

Our beliefs and values are synergistically linked.

Robert Dilts, an author and professor, adapted collective behavioral science studies to create what he calls the Logical Levels of Change.[50] While there are multiple steps in this model of behavior, the three I'd like to highlight here are:

Behaviors → Beliefs & Values → IDENTITY

Understanding the flow of these steps helps us to grasp the influence they have on each other. Our behaviors modify and influence our beliefs and values. Our beliefs and values then modify and influence our sense of identity.

Once repetition affirms a behavior, it has the power to change or add to our values and core beliefs. From there, we transform and revise our inner selves; ***we change who we are.***

---

50   https://www.logicallevels.co.uk/pages/logical-levels-model

You may recall the "two-word fix" mentioned in Chapter 18 of *Get Back into Whack*. I suggest swapping "I can't" to "I don't" (i.e., "I don't smoke" rather than "I can't smoke"). This switch helps us speak from a place of empowerment.

This week's theme gives you a broader understanding of why this is so. Empowered language comes from a shift in identity. Defining yourself as a non-smoker (or a non-junk food eater, etc.) is a claim of identity.

Can you feel the power of claiming something as who you are rather than just as something you do?

In Chapter 6 of *Get Back into Whack*, I shared why it's so important to use caution and care when choosing the words to use after an "I am" statement. The words that follow define *who* you believe you are. Imagine saying this, "I'm not good with numbers and find lots of ways to avoid getting my work reports done." It may sound like a simple reflection of a work problem. But let's be clear. If you said this, you'd have declared yourself to be a math-challenged procrastinator. There is a difference between a behavior and an identity. You may have circumstances where you struggle with math, but it's not *who* you are. You may struggle to get things done, but claiming the identity of a procrastinator does not serve you in any helpful way.

For the week ahead, pay attention to claims you make about who you are. Pay attention to identity statements, as well as your beliefs. One of the most empowering discoveries in the self-help or personal-development world is that your sense of identity can transform as you grow.

Who you are is not engraved in stone. Your behaviors, beliefs, and your identity are each malleable.

The choice is yours. Who do you want to be? Once you decide, evaluate what must happen for that to come true. What behaviors and beliefs would have to be in place first?

> ***"You have to be willing to go to war with yourself***
> ***and create a whole new identity."***
> —David Goggins

While the gist of this quote is accurate, I include it here for a specific reason. I want to point out the critical thinking error it contains.

I don't buy the part about war. Learning more about who we are and what makes us tick is an exploration of reflection, kindness, self-compassion, and acceptance. To me, anything contrary to that isn't about learning at all.

Is it time to put down your weapons and stop waging war at yourself?

SECTION NOTES:

SUMMARY:

H ealing is a process. It's a mission for both the body AND mind—a full-body experience. We could no more eat or exercise our way out of chronic illness than we could think our way out.

This workbook guides you on this healing path. In it, you'll find the themes necessary to build your mental, as well as physical muscles.

Are you setting yourself up for success by reviewing your mental movie of what you want from life right before you fall asleep? Are you mentally reviewing how you want your day to flow first thing as you wake? Are you priming your brain daily with encouraging thoughts, words, and images?

If so, here are some of the "side effects" you may experience:

- Positive shifts in the dominant emotions that come from your thoughts.
- Noticing that you automatically practice deep breathing, Tapping, or other effective stress management techniques in times of need.
- Noticing a shift in the "weight" of negative feelings and the lightness of positive ones.
- A natural desire to move your body in healthy ways.
- Natural changes in what you eat and what feels nourishing to your body.
- Feeling a partnership with those around you.
- Feeling a sense of peace and calm where there was once anxiety and overwhelm.
- Improved cognitive function, including memory and recall.

- An improved ability to apply self-compassion.
- Improved ability to fall asleep, stay asleep, and experience higher sleep quality.

Through the application of the themes outlined in this workbook, you'll experience improved brain health and function.[51]

What happens next?

Once you finish the practices from Week 12 of this workbook … flip back and start again! Revisit the healing themes from the beginning of Section 2 and zip through the 90-day program again. This time, use a different colored pen or pencil to jot down your notes.

As you work through the pages, notice how the application of time and experience modifies your perspective on the topics at hand. Some shifts may be nuanced and others profound. Zero in on the feelings and emotions of alignment. What feels right to you? Become curious. Investigate and consider new ideas as you layer in more changes for your mapped out future.

> *"Don't go through life; GROW through life."*
> — Eric Butterworth

Now you're equipped.
Design the life YOU desire!

---

51   https://www.forbes.com/sites/alicegwalton/2015/02/09/7-ways-meditation-can-actually-change-the-brain/#48c45c0b1465

RESOURCES GUIDE:

....

Please note that for strategic online marketing purposes, nearly all of my articles include fibromyalgia and/or chronic illness in the titles. That's my personal experience. ***It doesn't have to be yours.***

I don't want you to miss out on the value of these resources.

If fibromyalgia or chronic illness doesn't apply to you, that's okay. No matter what health or personal lifestyle challenge you're facing, you can find value in the resources offered here. If you'd like to feel better tomorrow than you do today, put into practice the essential tips, strategies, and ideas provided in the articles below.

Deep Breathing:
....

This Deep Breathing Calms Stress
https://rebuildingwellness.com/deep-breathing-chronic/

Relaxation Basics for Fibromyalgia and Chronic Illness
https://rebuildingwellness.com/relaxation-basics-fibromyalgia/

5 Fibro Stress Strategies
https://rebuildingwellness.com/5-fibro-stress-strategies/

Pathways Pain Relief for Fibromyalgia
https://rebuildingwellness.com/pathways-pain-fibro/

Gratitude:

Talk to Yourself and Make it Worthwhile
https://rebuildingwellness.com/talk-to-yourself/

Do You Want a Grateful Brain?
https://rebuildingwellness.com/do-you-want-a-grateful-brain/

The Power of the Pen
https://rebuildingwellness.com/the-power-of-the-pen/

Greens:

6 Ways Leafy Greens Heal Chronic Illness
https://rebuildingwellness.com/greens-heal-chronic-illness/

Try This Fast and Easy Nutritional Boost Today
https://rebuildingwellness.com/nutritional-boost/

Protein Green Smoothies
https://rebuildingwellness.com/protein-green-smoothies/

Simple Steps to Wellness
https://www.softsurroundings.com/blog/2012/10/05/simple-steps-to-wellness/

Healing Words:

The Fibro Brain and Healing Hopeful Words
https://rebuildingwellness.com/fibro-brain-words/

Rehearsing Positivity
https://rebuildingwellness.com/rehearsing-positivity/

4 Simple Ways to Shift into Positivity
https://www.prohealth.com/library/4-simple-ways-to-shift-into-positivity-6471

The Fibromyalgia Don't Do List
https://rebuildingwellness.com/fibromyalgia-dont-do-list/

Gut Connection to Intuitive Happiness
https://rebuildingwellness.com/gut-intuitive-happiness/

Putting a Stop to Negative Thoughts
https://rebuildingwellness.com/putting-a-stop-to-negative-thoughts/

Hydration:

Downloadable Water Hydration Tip Sheet for You!
https://rebuildingwellness.com/water-hydration-tip-sheet/

Fibromyalgia Struggles and How to Heal
https://rebuildingwellness.com/fibromyalgia-struggles-heal/

Motivation:

How to Get 3 Times the Motivation to Reach Your Goals
https://rebuildingwellness.com/get-3-times-motivation-goals/

Motivation: How to Create It
https://rebuildingwellness.com/create-motivation/

Lack Motivation? Plug into Your Core Values!
https://rebuildingwellness.com/motivation-core-values/

Moving Meditations:

Does Fibro Friendly Fitness Exist?
https://rebuildingwellness.com/fibro-aqua-therapy/

Gentle Healing with QiGong
https://rebuildingwellness.com/qigong/

Self-Care Must for Fibro
https://rebuildingwellness.com/self-care-must-fibro/

Moving Meditations for Chronic Healing
https://www.prohealth.com/library/moving-meditations-chronic-healing-86606

Rebuilding Wellness: One Person at a Time
https://www.prohealth.com/library/rebuilding-wellness-one-person-at-a-time-30980

Weight Loss, Fibromyalgia, and Fixes
https://rebuildingwellness.com/weight-loss-fibromyalgia-fixes/

Self-Care:
....

Self-care Must for Fibro
https://rebuildingwellness.com/self-care-must-fibro/

Self-care Results for Fibro
https://rebuildingwellness.com/self-care-results-fibro/

Tapping:
....

Tapping Key for Chronic Pain and Fibromyalgia
https://rebuildingwellness.com/tapping-fibromyalgia/

Tapping—a Somatic Approach to Fibromyalgia Pain
https://rebuildingwellness.com/tapping-somatic-fibro-pain/

Tapping into Healing Success with EFT
https://rebuildingwellness.com/tapping-healing-success-eft/

Values:

Healthy Changes and Your Core Values
https://rebuildingwellness.com/core-values/

Lack Motivation? Plug Into Your Core Values
https://rebuildingwellness.com/motivation-core-values/

Yoga:

Doable Yoga for Fibromyalgia
https://rebuildingwellness.com/doable-yoga-for-fibromyalgia/

Weight Loss, Fibromyalgia, and Fixes
https://rebuildingwellness.com/weight-loss-fibromyalgia-fixes/

LET'S GET CONNECTED!

 Follow my blog: https://www.rebuildingwellness.com/blog

 Facebook: https://www.facebook.com/pg/FibroWHYalgia/

 Twitter: https://twitter.com/sueinge

 Pinterest: https://www.pinterest.com/sueinge/

 Instagram: https://www.instagram.com/sue.ingebretson/

 LinkedIn: https://www.linkedin.com/in/sueinge/

ABOUT THE AUTHOR

Sue Ingebretson is a much sought after symptom-relief expert in the fibromyalgia, chronic illness, and autoimmune communities. Known for getting to the root of health challenges, her methods deliver long-term results using a light-hearted approach without quick-fix remedies that only mask symptoms.

She's an author, speaker, certified nutritional therapist, clinical hypnotherapist, master NLP practitioner, and an integrative nutrition health coach. She has additional certifications which include EFT, Time Line Therapy,® and Success Coaching. She leads workshops and seminars and writes for various in print and online publications.

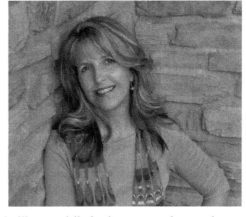

Her #1 Amazon bestselling book, *FibroWHYalgia* details her personal healing journey. Her activity book, *Chronic Coloring*, features fun, informative, and creative stress management solutions. Her newest books, *Get Back into Whack* and *Get Back into Whack Workbook* detail the brain's role in healing chronic illness while laying out a plan to do so.

Sue has been featured in *FIRST for Women* magazine, TV, ABC radio, and podcasts. She's active on a wide variety of social media platforms, and her blog with 500+ posts can be found at www. RebuildingWellness.com/blog.

About Rebuilding Wellness

Sue's life was out of control. She suffered from more symptoms than she could even list. She saw more than a dozen doctors who prescribed double that number of prescriptions.

She tried them all.

Finding no solutions, she took matters into her own hands and figured it out herself. Applying holistic healing and natural methods, she discovered what works best with the greatest economy and efficiency. It took time, tenacity, and a willingness to try new things to climb out of the pit from chronic illness to chronic wellness. But she's grateful for the journey.

Today, Sue encourages others to do the same—without the difficulties of going it alone. Seeded with light-hearted humor and support, she leads others (mostly women) through a step-by-step protocol designed to help them leave limiting symptoms behind and move toward a healthier and happier lifestyle. Want to learn more? Contact her here: http://rebuildingwellness.com/contact.

NOTES:

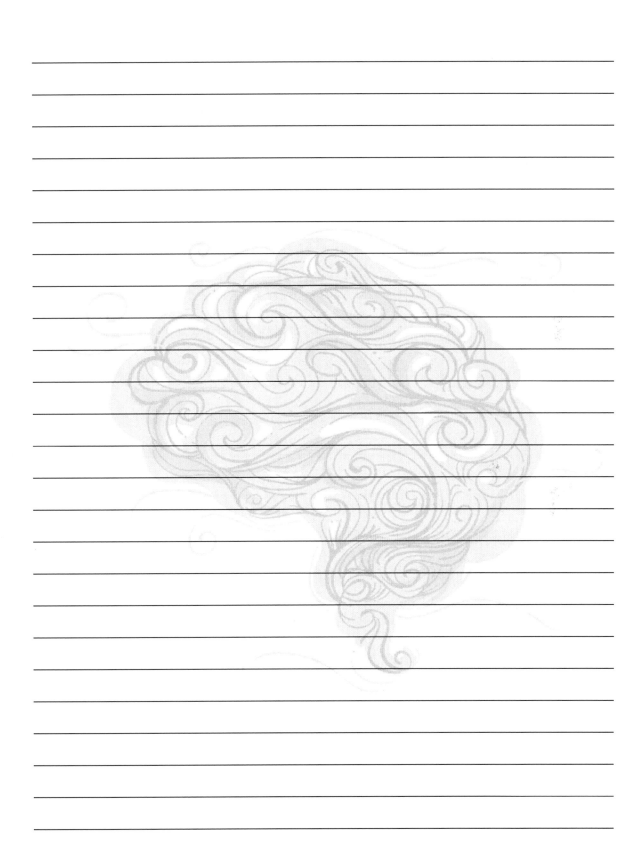

Printed in Great Britain
by Amazon